I0841559

Jet Set Pets

The Ultimate Guide to Traveling with Your Companion

M.A. Gorre

Copyright © 2023 by Michael Gorre

All rights reserved.

No portion of this book may be reproduced without written permission from the publisher or author except as permitted by U.S. copyright law.

Contents

Introduction

♥

Why This Book Matters

Traveling is one of life's great pleasures, and it becomes even more rewarding when you can share those experiences with your four-legged friend or feathered companion. Yet the idea of traveling with a pet can be daunting. Different regulations, the health of your pet, transportation options—all of these elements can make even the most organized person feel overwhelmed. This book aims to simplify that process, giving you a comprehensive guide that answers every question you might have. From airline regulations and road trip tips to international travel and finding pet-friendly accommodations, this book is designed to make traveling with your pet a breeze.

What to Expect

This book is structured to guide you through every stage of traveling with your pet, from preparation to your return home. Part I will walk you through the essential steps of preparing for your journey, including what to pack and how to get your pet ready for travel. Part II focuses exclusively on air travel, breaking down the complicated web of airline rules and regulations into easy-to-understand advice. For those hitting the road, Part III offers extensive tips on ensuring a safe and enjoyable road trip. Part IV addresses the complexities of international travel, including dealing with quarantine and understanding foreign pet regulations. Part V discusses accommodations and activities, while Part VI delves into safety and health considerations. Finally, Part VII will guide you through the steps you need to take when you and your pet return home.

Throughout the book, you'll find real-life examples, checklists, and practical advice to make your travels as smooth as possible. Whether you're flying across the world or just taking a weekend getaway, this book is your ultimate resource.

Your Ultimate Checklist for Traveling with Pets

Pre-Travel

- Vet visit for health check-up and vaccinations

- Research on airline/destination-specific regulations

- Purchase or check the condition of your pet carrier

- Compile all necessary travel paperwork (e.g., pet passport, permits)

- Create a packing list including food, snacks, toys, and first-aid supplies

During Travel

- Secure your pet in their carrier

- Keep important paperwork accessible

- Maintain feeding and hydration schedule

- Regular breaks for exercise and bathroom (if applicable)

Accommodations

- Confirm pet-friendly facilities

- Prepare a pet emergency kit

- Scout locations for outdoor activities and pet-friendly dining

Post-Travel

- Post-trip vet check-up

- Review your travel experience to improve future trips

- Properly store or dispose of any leftover travel supplies

This checklist serves as a quick reference guide and will be elaborated on in each relevant chapter. Keep it handy, and use it to ensure that you're fully prepared for an exciting and stress-free journey with your pet.

Preparing for the Journey

♥

The Essentials: What You Absolutely Need

When you're embarking on a journey, whether it's a short weekend getaway or a long overseas adventure, there's a lot to consider. But when you're traveling with a pet, those considerations multiply. After all, you're not just responsible for yourself but also for the well-being of your animal companion. In this chapter, we'll look at the fundamental essentials you absolutely need for pet travel. Having these essentials in place will help ensure a smooth, stress-free trip for both you and your pet.

Identification

First and foremost, your pet should have proper identification. This includes a collar with an ID tag that contains your contact information. The ID should include your name, phone number, and ideally, your travel destination. This will make it much easier for someone to contact you if your pet becomes lost.

Microchipping your pet is another crucial step. A microchip is a small implant that's placed under your pet's skin, usually between the shoulder blades. It contains a unique identification number linked to your contact information. In the event that your pet gets lost and is found by a vet or animal control, a quick scan of the chip will provide them with all the information they need to get in touch with you.

Vaccinations and Health Records

Before you travel, a trip to the vet is a must. Make sure your pet's vaccinations are up-to-date and request a health certificate dated within ten days of your departure. Some destinations, particularly international ones, have strict health requirements for animals. Without this certificate, your pet may be denied entry or subjected to quarantine.

Medications

If your pet is on any medications, bring enough to last the duration of your trip, plus a few extra days' worth in case of delays. This includes prescription medications, flea and tick treatments, and any over-the-counter remedies you use regularly.

Food and Water

You'll need to bring enough food to last for the entire trip, plus a little extra for emergencies. Make sure to also bring a portable water bowl and bottled water. Some pets can be sensitive to changes in water from different areas, which can lead to digestive issues.

Comfort Items

To help your pet adjust to new environments, bring along some comfort items like a favorite toy, blanket, or a piece of your clothing. These familiar items can help reduce your pet's stress and anxiety during travel.

First-Aid Kit

A basic pet first-aid kit is a must-have. This should include antiseptic wipes, gauze, bandages, and any other first-aid supplies recommended by your vet. You never know when an emergency will arise, so it's best to be prepared.

Choosing the Right Pet Carrier

Once you've covered the basic essentials, your next major consideration should be the pet carrier. This isn't just about picking something you think looks comfortable or secure. There are specific requirements, especially if you're planning to travel by air. Additionally, the right carrier can make all the difference in your pet's comfort and safety.

Size Matters

The carrier should be spacious enough for your pet to stand, turn around, and lie down comfortably. However, it shouldn't be so large that they slide around during transport. Airlines often have strict size requirements for carriers, so make sure you check those in advance.

Material and Construction

There are two main types of carriers: soft-sided and hard-sided. Soft-sided carriers are generally better for car travel and short trips. They are easier to carry and can fit more comfortably in various spaces. However, for air travel and long journeys, hard-sided carriers are recommended for their durability and structure. These carriers are usually made of hard plastic and offer better protection.

Ventilation

Good ventilation is essential, especially for long trips. Make sure the carrier has plenty of mesh panels or ventilation holes. This ensures that your pet will get enough fresh air and can also help reduce anxiety, as your pet can see its surroundings.

Accessibility

Opt for a carrier that has multiple entry and exit points. This makes it easier to get your pet in and out, especially in stressful or cramped situations.

Security

Zippers and locks should be of high quality to ensure that your pet can't escape during travel. Some carriers come with seatbelt loops, allowing you to secure the carrier in your car, which adds an extra layer of safety.

Special Features

Some carriers come with built-in compartments where you can store food, water, and other essentials. Others have attachable wheels or can convert into a backpack or rolling case. Think about your travel needs and whether these features would be useful for you.

Testing the Carrier

Before you embark on your journey, do some test runs with the carrier. Put your pet inside and go for a short drive or even a walk around the house. This helps your pet get accustomed to the carrier and allows you to see if there are any issues you hadn't considered.

By thoughtfully selecting a carrier and ensuring you have all the essential items, you're already well on your way to a successful journey with your pet. The right preparations can make the experience enjoyable and rewarding, allowing you both to make the most of your time away from home.

Visit the Vet: Health Checks and Vaccinations

One of the most critical steps before embarking on any journey with your pet is a visit to the veterinarian. This visit serves multiple purposes and ensures that your pet is in optimal health for travel. Here's what you need to cover:

Basic Health Check

Your vet will typically conduct a thorough examination to make sure there are no underlying health issues that could worsen while traveling. This will include checking your pet's weight, temperature, eyes, ears, and teeth.

Vaccinations

It's crucial to ensure that all vaccinations are up-to-date. Some destinations require specific vaccinations for pets, so discuss your travel plans with your vet to ensure you meet all requirements. Rabies, Bordetella, and distemper are some common vaccinations often needed.

Medication and Prescriptions

If your pet requires any medications, now is the time to refill those prescriptions. Ask your vet about any additional medications you might need for the trip, such as anti-anxiety meds or anti-nausea pills for pets prone to motion sickness.

Travel-Specific Health Certificate

Many places, especially international destinations, require a health certificate issued by a vet, usually within a specific time frame before travel. Make sure you know what's required and plan your vet visit accordingly.

Handling Anxiety:Both Yours and Your Pet's

Traveling can be stressful, both for humans and their animal companions. Here are some strategies to help you both cope:

For Your Pet

- **Familiarity**: Make sure to bring familiar items like your pet's blanket, toy, or even a piece of your clothing to comfort them.

- **Trial Runs**: Before the actual travel date, take short trips with your pet in their carrier to get them acclimated to the experience.

- **Anti-Anxiety Treats and Medication**: Some pets benefit from calming treats or even prescription anti-anxiety medication. Discuss options with your vet.

For You

- **Preparation**: The more you prepare, the less stressed you'll be. Make checklists, pack well in advance, and confirm all arrangements ahead of time.

- **Breathing Exercises**: Techniques such as deep breathing can help calm nerves.

- **Stay Calm**: Pets pick up on human emotions. The calmer you are, the more likely your pet will also remain calm

Travel Paperwork: Permits, Passports, and More

Regulations can vary dramatically depending on your destination. Here's what you might need:

- **Pet Passport**: In some places like the European Union, a pet passport that includes details of vaccinations and microchipping is required.

- **Permits**: Some destinations require a permit for pets, which must be applied for well in advance.

- **Health Certificate**: As mentioned earlier, many places require a certificate from a vet confirming your pet is fit to travel.

- **Quarantine Information**: Research if your destination requires a quarantine period for arriving pets and prepare accordingly.

Visit the Vet: Health Check and Vaccinations

♥

One of the most critical steps before embarking on any journey with your pet is a visit to the veterinarian. This visit serves multiple purposes and ensures that your pet is in optimal health for travel. Here's what you need to cover:

Basic Health Check

Your vet will typically conduct a thorough examination to make sure there are no underlying health issues that could worsen while traveling. This will include checking your pet's weight, temperature, eyes, ears, and teeth.

Vaccinations

It's crucial to ensure that all vaccinations are up-to-date. Some destinations require specific vaccinations for pets, so discuss your travel plans with your vet to ensure you meet all requirements. Rabies, Bordetella, and distemper are some common vaccinations often needed.

Medication and Prescriptions

If your pet requires any medications, now is the time to refill those prescriptions. Ask your vet about any additional medications you might need for the trip, such as anti-anxiety meds or anti-nausea pills for pets prone to motion sickness.

Travel-Specific Health Certificate

Many places, especially international destinations, require a health certificate issued by a vet, usually within a specific time frame before travel. Make sure you know what's required and plan your vet visit accordingly.

Handling Anxiety: Both Yours and Your Pet's

Traveling can be stressful, both for humans and their animal companions. Here are some strategies to help you both cope:

For Your Pet

- **Familiarity**: Make sure to bring familiar items like your pet's blanket, toy, or even a piece of your clothing to comfort them.

- **Trial Runs**: Before the actual travel date, take short trips with your pet in their carrier to get them acclimated to the experience.

- **Anti-Anxiety Treats and Medication**: Some pets benefit from calming treats or even prescription anti-anxiety medication. Discuss options with your vet.

For You

- **Preparation**: The more you prepare, the less stressed you'll be. Make checklists, pack well in advance, and confirm all arrangements ahead of time.

- **Breathing Exercises**: Techniques such as deep breathing can help calm nerves.

- **Stay Calm**: Pets pick up on human emotions. The calmer you are, the more likely your pet will also remain calm.

Travel Paperwork: Permits, Passports, and More

Regulations can vary dramatically depending on your destination. Here's what you might need:

- **Pet Passport**: In some places like the European Union, a pet passport that includes details of vaccinations and microchipping is required.

- **Permits**: Some destinations require a permit for pets, which must be applied for well in advance.

- **Health Certificate**: As mentioned earlier, many places require a certificate from a vet confirming your pet is fit to travel.

- **Quarantine Information**: Research if your destination requires a quarantine period for arriving pets and prepare accordingly.

Food, Snacks, and Hydration: What to Pack

- **Dry Food**: Easier to pack and less prone to spoilage.

- **Canned Food**: If your pet usually eats canned food, bring a few cans along with a way to reseal them.

- **Treats**: Great for rewarding good behavior and for training purposes.

- **Water**: Bring bottled water and a portable bowl for your pet.

- **Special Diets**: If your pet has specific dietary needs, make sure to pack sufficient supplies.

Training Your Pet for Travel

If your pet isn't used to traveling, then it's a good idea to get them acclimated before the big trip. Here's how:

- **Carrier Training**: Encourage your pet to spend time in their carrier by placing treats or toys inside.

- **Car Training**: Take your pet on short car rides, gradually increasing the time spent in the vehicle.

- **Socialization**: Expose your pet to new experiences, people, and other animals to prepare them for new encounters they might have during the trip.

- **Command Training**: Ensure your pet understands basic commands like "stay," "come," and "sit." This will be invaluable in keeping them safe and well-behaved during your travels.

Taking the time to prepare for your journey can make all the difference in the world, making the trip more enjoyable and less stressful for both you and your pet.

Airline Travel

Travelling by air with a pet presents its own unique set of challenges. From airline-specific regulations to ensuring your pet's comfort and safety during the flight, there's a lot to consider. This chapter aims to demystify the process and offer you a roadmap for navigating air travel with your pet successfully.

Researching Pet-Friendly Airlines

Not all airlines are created equal when it comes to pet travel, and the differences can be substantial. Here's what to consider when researching pet-friendly airlines:

Cabin or Cargo?

The most significant decision you'll likely make is whether your pet will travel in the cabin with you or in the cargo hold. Most airlines allow small pets in the cabin for an additional fee, but size restrictions apply. Larger animals typically have to travel in the cargo hold, which is temperature-controlled but can be more stressful for the pet.

Airline Pet Policies

Each airline has its own pet policy, including rules about the type, size, and breed of pets they allow. Some airlines also have restrictions on how many pets can travel in the cabin per flight, so it's advisable to book early.

Fees and Costs

Costs can vary widely from one airline to the next. Some airlines charge a flat fee for pet travel, while others may charge based on the pet's size or weight. Always read the fine print to understand what you're paying for.

Reviews and Testimonials

It's always a good idea to read reviews from other pet owners who have traveled with the airline you're considering. Personal experiences can offer invaluable insights into how well an airline accommodates pets.

International Travel

If you're traveling internationally, the airline you choose needs to comply with the pet import regulations of your destination country. This often involves coordinating with local animal control or quarantine facilities, so it's crucial to choose an airline experienced in international pet travel.

Special Needs

If your pet has specific medical or emotional needs, consult with the airline to see how they can accommodate these. Some airlines offer specialized services for pets with anxiety, mobility issues, or medical needs.

Layovers and Extended Travel

If your travel involves layovers, consider how this will affect your pet. It's always best to choose the most direct route possible to minimize stress and potential complications for your pet. Some airports have pet-relief areas where you can take your pet during layovers, and a few even offer pet care facilities where your pet can be fed and exercised during extended layovers.

By doing thorough research, you can ensure that you choose the best airline for both you and your pet, making the journey as smooth and comfortable as possible. It takes time and effort to sift through the various policies and reviews, but the peace of mind you'll gain is well worth the investment.

Understanding Airline Policies

Before you book a flight for you and your pet, you'll need to become well-versed in your chosen airline's pet policies. Each airline has its unique set of guidelines, and failing to adhere to them could result in a stressful experience or even denial of boarding. Here are key points to look for when understanding airline policies:

Pet Carrier Specifications

Airlines have strict rules about the size and type of pet carriers they allow. Make sure your carrier complies with these specifications, or you might be required to purchase an airline-approved carrier at the airport, which can be quite expensive.

Documentation

Certain airlines require specific documentation, such as a health certificate or proof of vaccinations, to be presented at the time of check-in or before boarding. Know what paperwork you'll need to have on hand.

Restricted Breeds

Some airlines have breed restrictions, particularly for brachycephalic breeds (like pugs and bulldogs), which are prone to respiratory issues. Make sure your pet's breed is not on the airline's restricted list.

In-Cabin vs. Cargo Hold

Find out whether your pet is eligible to travel in the cabin or must be placed in the cargo hold. This often depends on your pet's size and the airline's specific policies.

Age Restrictions

Some airlines have age requirements for pets, often requiring them to be at least eight weeks old. This is particularly common for puppies and kittens.

Fee Structure

Fully understand the airline's fee structure for traveling with a pet, as these can vary. Some airlines charge per leg of the journey, while others charge a flat rate.

Emergency Protocols

Know what the airline's protocols are in case of an emergency, such as a medical issue with your pet during the flight. This information is usually available on the airline's website or through customer service.

Booking the Ticket: Direct Flight vs. Layover

When it comes to pet travel, the type of flight you choose can make a significant difference in your pet's overall experience and comfort. Here's what to consider:

Direct Flight

- **Advantages**: A direct flight is often the best option when traveling with a pet. It minimizes the amount of time your pet spends in the carrier and reduces the risk of mishandling during layovers.

- **Disadvantages**: Direct flights can be more expensive and might not be available for all destinations.

Layover

- **Advantages**: Flights with layovers can be less expensive and may offer more flexible scheduling options.

- **Disadvantages**: Layovers increase the total travel time and can be stressful for your pet. There's also a higher risk of delays or complications, such as missed connections, which can be particularly problematic when traveling with a pet.

Key Considerations

- **Pet Relief Areas**: If a layover is unavoidable, look for airports that offer pet relief areas where you can let your pet stretch and relieve themselves during the layover.

- **Layover Duration**: A longer layover may provide an opportunity for you to spend some time with your pet, but it also prolongs the overall travel time. Choose wisely based on your pet's temperament and needs.

By fully understanding airline policies and carefully considering your flight options, you can make informed decisions that will help ensure a smooth and comfortable travel experience for both you and your pet.

Pre-Flight Preparations

♥

Preparing for a flight with your pet involves more than just packing a bag and heading to the airport. There are several steps you should take in the days and hours leading up to your flight to ensure that both you and your pet have a smooth travel experience. Here are some key pre-flight preparations:

Final Vet Visit

Schedule a final check-up with your veterinarian a few days before your trip to ensure all vaccinations are up-to-date and you have all necessary health certificates and medications.

Pet Identification

Make sure your pet's ID tags are current and securely attached to their collar. Consider a temporary travel tag with your contact information at your destination.

Packing Essentials

Double-check your packing list to ensure you have all the essentials your pet will need, including food, water, leash, waste bags, and any medications or comfort items.

Pre-Flight Meal

Feed your pet a light meal 3 to 4 hours before departure. Avoid feeding right before the flight to minimize the risk of stomach upset during the flight.

Exercise

Give your pet plenty of exercise before heading to the airport to help them burn off excess energy and hopefully make them a bit tired for the journey.

Airport Security: A Step-by-Step Guide

Navigating airport security can be one of the most stressful aspects of traveling with a pet. Knowing what to expect and how best to prepare can help alleviate some of this stress. Here's a step-by-step guide to help you through the process:

Arrival and Check-In

- **Early Arrival**: Arrive at the airport at least 2 hours before a domestic flight and 3 hours for international flights to allow time for any unexpected delays during the check-in and security processes.

- **Documentation**: Have all required documents such as your pet's health certificate, proof of vaccinations, and any necessary permits easily accessible.

The Security Line

- **Pet Carrier**: Your pet will need to be removed from its carrier, which will go through the X-ray machine.

- **Leash**: Keep a leash handy to control your pet while you both go through security. Some airports have a separate screening process for pets, but often you'll simply walk your pet through the metal detector while holding them or on a leash.

Personal Screening

- **Pet Handling**: You will need to hold your pet or have them on a leash while you undergo any additional screening.

- **Secondary Inspection**: In some cases, security personnel may request a secondary inspection of your pet or their carrier. Follow all instructions and remain calm to help your pet stay calm too.

Post-Security

- **Repack**: Once you've cleared security, repack any items that were removed from your pet's carrier and ensure they are safely enclosed before heading to your departure gate.

- **Relax**: Take some time to let your pet drink some water and relax a bit before boarding the flight.

Understanding the pre-flight and airport security procedures can make the process smoother and less stressful for both you and your pet. With adequate preparation, your journey can be as hassle-free as possible, setting the stage for a successful trip.

In-Flight Tips and Etiquette

♥

Once you've made it through airport security and boarded the plane, you might think the hard part is over. However, flying can be a stressful experience for pets, so it's crucial to be prepared and know how to make the flight as comfortable as possible for your furry companion. Here's a guide to in-flight tips and etiquette to ensure a smooth journey for everyone involved.

Comfort and Safety

Proper Positioning

Place your pet's carrier under the seat in front of you if they are traveling in the cabin. Follow the airline's guidelines for pets traveling in the cargo hold, ensuring they are properly secured.

Keep Calm

Your pet will likely sense your emotions, so it's important to stay calm. Speak softly to your pet, and avoid fussing or showing signs of anxiety, as it can make them more nervous.

Minimize Movement

Try to stay in your seat as much as possible to reduce disruption for other passengers and to keep your pet's environment stable.

Feeding and Hydration

Water

Offer your pet small amounts of water periodically to keep them hydrated, but not so much that it might upset their stomach.

Snacks

If it's a long flight, you can offer a small snack or two, but avoid feeding a full meal until you arrive at your destination.

Bathroom Needs

Absorbent Pad

Place an absorbent pad in your pet's carrier in case of accidents. Some airlines also offer "pet relief areas" inside the aircraft for long-haul flights.

Holding It

Train your pet to "hold it" for extended periods before the flight. Most domestic flights are short enough that this won't be an issue, but it's something to consider for longer journeys.

Social Etiquette

Quiet Time

Encourage your pet to be as quiet as possible. Bring along their favorite toy or blanket to help comfort them and keep them occupied.

Interactions with Other Passengers

Be considerate of other passengers by minimizing any disruptions your pet may cause. If your pet is anxious or making noise, try to soothe them quietly and efficiently.

Cabin Crew Instructions

Always listen to the cabin crew's instructions regarding pet travel. They are trained to handle a variety of situations and their guidance is crucial for everyone's safety and comfort.

By following these in-flight tips and etiquette guidelines, you can contribute to a more peaceful and comfortable experience for you, your pet, and your fellow passengers. Safe travels!

Surviving Layovers and Transits

♥

If your journey involves layovers or transits, additional challenges come into play when you're traveling with a pet. This section offers practical advice on how to make this experience less stressful for both you and your furry friend.

Planning Your Route

Shortest Layover Possible

A shorter layover minimizes the time your pet spends confined in their carrier, but make sure you have enough time to attend to your pet's needs and make it to your next flight.

Pet-Friendly Airports

Whenever possible, choose airports known for their pet-friendly facilities. Some airports have designated pet relief areas and even pet lounges where your pet can stretch and relieve themselves.

Timing

Avoid layovers during extreme weather conditions, be it heat or cold, especially if your pet will be traveling in the cargo hold. This will help ensure their comfort and safety.

During the Layover

Check on Your Pet

If your pet is traveling in the cargo hold, some airlines allow you to check on them during long layovers. Verify this option in advance.

Pet Relief Areas

Use pet relief areas if available. If not, find a quiet corner where you can lay down a pee pad for your pet.

Food and Water

Offer a small amount of food and water, but be cautious not to overfeed, as you don't want your pet to be uncomfortable on the next leg of the journey.

Exercise

Use any extra time to let your pet stretch their legs and expend some energy, which can be especially beneficial before boarding another flight.

Common Challenges and Solutions

Delays and Cancellations

Have a contingency plan in case of unexpected delays or cancellations. Keep extra food, water, and medication in your carry-on.

Behavioral Issues

If your pet is anxious or restless, use calming techniques such as petting, soft talking, or even a pet-calming spray or treat, if you have one.

Communication

Keep an open line of communication with airline staff, particularly if you have tight connections or special needs for your pet.

Arrival and Transition to Next Flight

Update Information

Check that your pet's tag or microchip information is correct and current, especially if you have multiple flights or airlines involved.

Final Check

Before boarding your next flight, ensure that your pet's carrier is secure and that they are comfortable and ready for the next part of the journey.

By anticipating potential challenges and knowing how to address them, you can make layovers and transits much more manageable experiences for both you and your pet. Proper planning and a little bit of foresight can go a long way in ensuring a smoother, less stressful journey.

Road Trips: Vehicle Safety for Pets

♥

Traveling with your pet by car offers more flexibility compared to air travel, but it comes with its own set of challenges and safety considerations. Whether you're going for a short drive to the vet or embarking on a cross-country adventure, ensuring your pet's safety and comfort in the vehicle is paramount. Below are tips and guidelines for vehicle safety for pets during road trips.

Before Hitting the Road

Vehicle Preparation

- Make sure the vehicle is clean and free of any hazardous objects that could harm your pet.

- Consider installing a pet barrier or seat protector to contain fur, dander, and possible accidents.

Trial Runs

- Before the actual trip, take a few short drives to help your pet acclimatize to car travel. Observe how they react and adjust your plans accordingly.

Packing Essentials

- Pack a travel kit that includes water, pet food, a leash, waste bags, medication, and any other necessities.

Securing Your Pet

Harnesses and Seat Belts

- The safest way for a dog to travel in a car is secured in a harness attached to a seat belt.

- For smaller pets like cats, a well-ventilated, secure carrier is advisable.

Pet Carriers

- If using a carrier, ensure it is stable and won't slide or tip over during the journey.

- Never put the carrier in the front seat, as airbags can seriously injure your pet in case of an accident.

Windows and Doors

- Always keep windows partially closed to prevent your pet from sticking its head out, as this can lead to injury.

- Use child locks to prevent your pet from accidentally opening windows or doors.

On The Road

Frequent Stops

- Plan for frequent stops to allow your pet to stretch, use the restroom, and hydrate.

Keep Them Inside

- Never leave your pet alone in a parked car, especially in hot or cold weather, as this can be life-threatening.

Air Conditioning and Ventilation

- Ensure proper ventilation and temperature control. If it's hot, use air conditioning; if it's cold, ensure the car is adequately heated.

Emergency Preparedness

First Aid Kit

- Keep a pet-specific first aid kit in the car for emergencies. This should include bandages, antiseptics, and any medication your pet might need.

Identification

- Make sure your pet's ID tags are up to date and securely fastened to their collar. Also, consider microchipping your pet as an added precaution.

Emergency Contacts

- Keep a list of emergency contact numbers, including your vet and nearby animal hospitals, readily accessible.

By adhering to these vehicle safety tips for pets, you can ensure that your road trip is enjoyable for both you and your furry companion. Preparation and awareness are key to a smooth and safe journey

Packing the Car: Room for Everyone

♥

Successfully packing the car for a road trip involves striking the right balance between accommodating everyone's needs and making efficient use of space. When traveling with pets, this becomes especially important. Here's a guide to help you pack your car in a way that ensures comfort and safety for all passengers, including your furry friend.

Planning the Layout

Prioritize Essentials

- Identify items you'll need easy access to, such as your pet's food, water, leash, and toys. Keep these within arm's reach.

Human vs. Pet Space

- Allocate sufficient space for both human passengers and pets. Cramped spaces can lead to stress and discomfort for everyone.

Safety Measures

- Use safety features like tie-downs or cargo nets to secure loose items that could shift during the drive and potentially cause harm.

Packing Order

Bottom Layer

- Start with heavier, rarely-needed items at the bottom, like spare tires, tools, and emergency kits.

Middle Layer

- Place mid-weight items such as suitcases and cooler boxes above the heavier layer, making sure they are stable.

Top Layer

- Lighter, frequently-used items like snack bags, pet treats, and first-aid kits should go on top for easy access.

Pet-Specific Packing

Pet Carrier or Harness

- Position your pet's carrier or harness so that it is easily accessible and well-ventilated. Avoid placing heavy items on or against it.

Pet Supplies

- Keep a small bag containing your pet's essentials—food, leash, waste bags—near the seat where you'll be sitting for quick access.

Double-Check for Safety

Unobstructed Views

- Ensure that your packing does not obstruct your views through any of the mirrors or windows.

Loose Items

- Secure any loose items that could become projectiles in case of sudden stops.

Accessibility

- Make sure human and pet passengers can easily get in and out of the car, especially for planned rest stops.

Quick Unpacking

Overnight Bag

- If your road trip spans multiple days, consider packing an overnight bag with essentials for both you and your pet to avoid unpacking the entire car at every stop.

By taking the time to carefully pack your car, you can ensure that both human and pet passengers have a comfortable and safe journey. Efficient packing allows for easier access to necessities, a less cluttered space, and, ultimately, a more enjoyable road trip for everyone.

On the Road: Stops, Rests, and Meals

♥

Long road trips require well-planned stops for rest, meals, and bathroom breaks—not just for humans but for our pets as well. Knowing how to effectively manage these stops can make the difference between a stressful journey and a pleasurable travel experience. Here's a comprehensive guide for making your stops as efficient and comfortable as possible.

Planning Your Stops

Schedule

- Aim to stop every 2-4 hours to allow everyone, including your pet, to stretch their legs and take a bathroom break.

Map Out Locations

- Use maps or apps to find pet-friendly rest areas, parks, or even specific restaurants where pets are welcome.

Weather Considerations

- Plan your stops based on the weather. For instance, if it's hot, look for shaded areas for breaks, and if it's cold, find spots where you can quickly get indoors.

Rest Stops

Exercise and Playtime

- Use this time to let your pet run around a little. A game of fetch can help them get rid of pent-up energy.

Potty Breaks

- Ensure that you clean up after your pet. Always carry a supply of waste bags for this purpose.

Snacks and Hydration

- Offer water and perhaps a small snack to your pet. However, avoid feeding them a full meal unless it's mealtime.

Meal Stops

Pet-Friendly Dining

- Opt for restaurants that have pet-friendly outdoor seating areas or get takeout that you can enjoy at a park or rest area with your pet.

Feeding Your Pet

- Serve your pet their meal in a collapsible dish or directly from their travel food container.

Avoid Human Food

- Resist the urge to share your food with your pet, especially foods that may be harmful to them, like chocolate, grapes, or anything with xylitol.

Health and Well-being

Check for Ticks

- If you've stopped in a wooded area or a place with tall grass, do a quick tick check on both yourself and your pet before getting back into the car.

Medication and Supplements

- If your pet is on medication or takes supplements, be sure to administer them according to the schedule.

Last-Minute Checks

Car Inspection

- Before heading back on the road, give your car a quick inspection to make sure everything is in order.

Pet's Comfort

- Ensure your pet is safely secured in their harness or carrier and seems comfortable and ready to continue the journey.

Planning and executing your stops thoughtfully can contribute to a successful road trip, making the journey enjoyable for everyone involved, including your pet. The key is to be organized, flexible, and considerate of your pet's needs.

Navigating Heavy Traffic

♥

Safe Distance

- Keep a safe distance from the vehicle in front of you to avoid sudden braking, which could disturb your pet.

Calming Techniques

- Heavy traffic can cause stress. Use calming techniques like playing soft music or speaking in a soothing tone to both yourself and your pet.

Ventilation

- In slow-moving traffic, make sure there is good air circulation to keep your pet comfortable.

Winding and Hilly Roads

Secure the Carrier

- Make sure the pet carrier is secure and won't slide or tip over during sharp turns or inclines.

Slow Down

- Take curves and steep roads at reduced speeds to minimize motion sickness for both humans and pets.

Frequent Stops

- Winding roads can be disorienting for pets. Take more frequent stops to let your pet regain their bearings.

Driving in Inclement Weather

Visibility

- Keep windows clear for maximum visibility. Use defoggers and wipers as needed.

Temperature Control

- Use air conditioning or heating to maintain a comfortable temperature for your pet.

Emergency Supplies

- Keep blankets, towels, and a first-aid kit handy in case of weather-related issues like mud, snow, or rain.

Unexpected Road Conditions

Detours and Delays

- Have a Plan B for your route in case of unexpected detours or road closures.

Roadside Assistance

- Keep numbers for roadside assistance handy, and make sure they are pet-friendly services in case you need a tow.

Survival Kit

- Always have an emergency survival kit that includes essentials for your pet like extra food, water, and medication.

By preparing for different traffic scenarios and road conditions, and by being vigilant while driving, you can make the journey safer and more comfortable for you and your pet. It takes a little extra effort, but the peace of mind it brings is well worth it.

Hotel Stays: Booking Pet-Friendly Accommodations

♥

Finding the right place to stay is crucial when you're traveling with your pet. Fortunately, Canada and the United States have a growing number of hotels that welcome four-legged guests. In this guide, we'll outline what to consider when booking pet-friendly accommodations and how to make your hotel stay as comfortable as possible for both you and your pet.

Research and Planning

Online Resources

- Use dedicated websites and apps that specialize in pet-friendly accommodations to search for hotels in your destination.

Reviews and Recommendations

- Read reviews from other pet owners to get an idea of how genuinely pet-friendly a hotel is.

Budget Considerations

- Keep in mind that some hotels charge a pet fee, which can range from a flat rate to a nightly charge.

Making Reservations

Call Ahead

- Always call the hotel directly to confirm that they can accommodate your pet, even if the website states that it is pet-friendly.

Specific Needs

- Discuss any specific requirements you may have, such as extra space for a large dog or a room away from high-traffic areas for a skittish pet.

Policies and Fees

- Familiarize yourself with the hotel's pet policies, including fees, restricted areas, and any weight or breed limitations.

Check-In

Paperwork

- You may need to sign a pet policy agreement upon arrival. Make sure to read this carefully.

Welcome Kit

- Some pet-friendly hotels offer a welcome kit that includes treats, a toy, and a list of local pet services, such as vets and pet stores.

During the Stay

Pet Etiquette

- Always keep your pet leashed or in a carrier in common areas, and adhere to any designated pet relief zones for bathroom breaks.

Housekeeping

- Use the "Do Not Disturb" sign when you leave your pet in the room or coordinate with housekeeping to clean when you're present.

Exercise

- Take advantage of any pet-friendly amenities, like a designated pet play area or nearby parks.

Check-Out

Inspect the Room

- Before leaving, inspect the room for any damage or forgotten items, like your pet's favorite toy.

Feedback and Reviews

- Provide feedback to the hotel, either directly or through an online review, to help them improve their pet-friendly services.

By following these tips and guidelines, you can ensure a comfortable and stress-free hotel stay for you and your pet. Whether you're traveling in Canada or the U.S., plenty of accommodations are willing to go the extra mile to make your furry companion feel at home.

International Travel with Pets

♥

Taking your pet across borders involves careful planning and an understanding of various regulations and requirements. Different countries have different rules about importing animals, and failing to comply can lead to delays, quarantine, or even denial of entry. This guide covers the essential aspects of international travel with your pet, including country-specific regulations and how to deal with quarantine procedures.

Country-Specific Regulations

Research and Documentation

- Before planning any international trip, research the pet import regulations of the country you'll be visiting. Requirements can include specific vaccinations, microchipping, and parasite treatments.

Consult Official Websites

- Government websites and consulate offices are the best sources for accurate and updated information on pet travel regulations.

Import Permits

- Some countries require an import permit for pets. The process to obtain this can be lengthy, so start well in advance of your travel date.

Breed Restrictions

- Note that some countries have restrictions on certain breeds. Make sure to check if your pet's breed is allowed in the country you're visiting.

Preparing for the Journey

Vet Visits

- Schedule a comprehensive health check-up for your pet, focusing on the specific vaccinations and tests required by the destination country.

International Health Certificates

- Most countries require a vet-issued International Health Certificate stating that the pet is fit for travel and meets all the health requirements of the destination country.

Language Barriers

- Translate all your pet's documents if you're traveling to a country where the official language is not English.

Dealing with Quarantine

Know the Rules

- Quarantine rules vary by country. Some have strict mandatory quarantine periods for incoming pets, while others have more lenient regulations if specific conditions are met.

Prepare Your Pet

- If your pet must undergo quarantine, help prepare them by gradually accustoming them to spending time in confined spaces.

Quarantine Facilities

- Research and visit the quarantine facilities if possible. Make sure they meet your standards for your pet's care and well-being.

Communication

- Stay in constant communication with the quarantine facility to monitor your pet's health and mental state during the separation period.

Arrival and Customs

Customs Declaration

- Upon arrival, you'll usually need to declare your pet at customs. Have all your paperwork organized and readily available.

Inspection

- Your pet might have to undergo an immediate health inspection. Keep any relevant health certificates and veterinary documents at hand for this process.

By diligently researching and preparing for the regulations and requirements of international pet travel, you can make the process much smoother for both you and your pet. Though the process may seem overwhelming, a well-planned trip can ensure that your pet is allowed to accompany you in your international adventures without any hiccups.

Customs and Import Regulations: Common Obstacles, and Budgeting for Your Trip

♥

Traveling internationally with your pet involves navigating through customs and import regulations, dealing with common obstacles, and carefully budgeting for all expected and unexpected expenses. Here's a guide that covers these three critical areas.

Customs and Import Regulations

Pet Import Forms

- Obtain and fill out any required pet import forms for the destination country, often available on the country's embassy or customs website.

Timing Is Everything

- Some countries require that specific forms be completed within a set period before your departure. Make sure to keep track of these deadlines.

Import Duties

- Some countries impose import duties on pets. Check in advance so you can budget accordingly.

Contraband Items

- Note that some pet supplies may not be allowed into the destination country. Research this in advance to avoid confiscation at the border.

Common Obstacles and How to Overcome Them

Flight Delays and Cancellations

- Plan for contingencies like flight delays or cancellations, which could affect your pet's feeding and medication schedules.

Solution

- Pack extra food and medicine in your carry-on and research pet-friendly accommodations near the airport.

Missing or Incorrect Paperwork

- Incomplete or incorrect paperwork can result in delays or even denial of entry for your pet.

Solution

- Double-check all paperwork for accuracy, and carry extra copies.

Language Barriers

- In countries where English is not the primary language, explaining your pet's needs can be challenging.

Solution

- Learn basic phrases related to pet care in the local language or use a translation app.

Currency and Costs: Budgeting for Your Trip

Currency Exchange Rates

- Be aware of currency exchange rates when budgeting for your trip. Fluctuations can impact your expenses.

Hidden Costs

- Beyond the obvious costs like flights and accommodation, remember to budget for pet fees, import duties, and emergency vet visits.

Travel Insurance

- Consider taking out travel insurance that covers pet emergencies. Read the fine print to make sure it provides adequate coverage.

Daily Budget

- Account for your pet's daily expenses like food, bottled water (if tap water isn't safe), and possibly even pet-sitting services if you plan to do activities where pets aren't allowed.

By being well-prepared and well-informed, you can mitigate many of the challenges associated with international pet travel. A well-planned budget will also help you avoid financial strain, ensuring that both you and your pet can enjoy the adventure without any added stress.

Accommodations and Activities: Researching Pet-Friendly Options and Weighing Airbnb vs. Hotels

♥

When traveling with your pet, choosing the right accommodation is crucial for a stress-free experience. Whether you're looking at Airbnb listings or traditional hotels, each has its pros and cons. This guide will help you navigate your options and find an environment where both you and your pet will be comfortable.

Researching Pet-Friendly Accommodations

Online Resources

- Utilize pet-specific travel websites and apps to find hotels, hostels, and Airbnb listings that are pet-friendly.

Reviews

- Read reviews left by other pet owners. They will often give you an idea of how welcoming and convenient the accommodation really is for pets.

Amenities

- Look for places that offer pet-friendly amenities like a fenced yard, pet bowls, or a pet play area.

Ask Directly

- When in doubt, reach out directly to the accommodation to inquire about their pet policy, any restrictions, and available amenities for pets.

Airbnb vs. Hotels: Pros and Cons

Airbnb: Pros

More Like Home

- Airbnb listings often offer a more home-like environment, which can be less stressful for pets.

Varied Options

- You can find listings with specific features like a backyard or a pet-friendly neighborhood.

Kitchen Access

- Having a kitchen allows you to prepare your pet's meals just like you would at home.

Airbnb: Cons

Inconsistent Policies

- Pet policies can vary greatly between listings. Always read the fine print.

No On-site Staff

- Lack of on-site staff means you're on your own for pet care and emergencies.

Security Deposit

- Some listings require a pet deposit, which could be costly.

Hotels: Pros

Consistency

- Chain hotels often have consistent pet policies, making it easier to know what to expect.

On-site Amenities

- Many hotels offer pet-specific amenities like dog-walking services or pet-sitting.

Immediate Assistance

- Hotels have staff that can assist with any pet-related emergencies or needs.

Hotels: Cons

Limited Space

- Hotels usually offer less space for pets to roam compared to Airbnb listings.

Extra Fees

- Many hotels charge a non-refundable pet fee on top of your booking cost.

Restrictions

- Hotels may have weight and breed restrictions, as well as limits on the number of pets allowed.

Choosing between Airbnb and a hotel ultimately depends on your specific needs, budget, and the kind of experience you want for yourself and your pet. Regardless of what you choose, thorough research and preparation are key to ensuring a smooth and enjoyable trip.

Parks, Trails, Outdoor Activities, and More:
A Guide to Pet-Friendly Entertainment and Dining

❤️

Traveling with your pet doesn't have to mean sacrificing your vacation experiences. Many destinations offer pet-friendly parks, trails, indoor entertainment options, and dining establishments. This guide will help you explore a variety of activities you can enjoy with your furry friend in tow.

Parks, Trails, and Outdoor Activities

Research Local Parks

- Use local tourism websites or apps like AllTrails to find nearby parks that welcome pets.

Dog Parks

- If your pet enjoys socializing, look for dog parks where they can run freely and interact with other dogs.

Beaches and Lakes

- Some locations offer pet-friendly beaches or lakefront areas. Always adhere to local guidelines about leashes and clean-up.

Hiking Trails

- Some trails are pet-friendly. Make sure to check if there are any restrictions, such as leash laws or areas where pets are not allowed.

Adventure Activities

- More adventurous? Some places offer pet-friendly kayaking, paddleboarding, or even zip-lining.

Indoor Entertainment: Pet-Friendly Places to Go

Pet-Friendly Museums and Galleries

- Some museums and art galleries allow pets. Check their websites or call ahead to confirm.

Shopping Centers

- Look for pet-friendly malls or shopping centers where dogs are welcome in common areas or certain stores.

Activity Centers

- Some cities have indoor play centers specifically designed for pets, complete with obstacle courses and toys.

Rainy Day Activities

- Bookstores, pet shops, and even some cafes offer a good retreat for a rainy day.

Dining Out: Pet-Friendly Restaurants and Cafés

Research Ahead of Time

- Use apps or websites like BringFido to find pet-friendly dining establishments.

Outdoor Seating

- Many restaurants with patios or beer gardens allow pets in their outdoor seating areas.

Pet Menus

- Some eateries go the extra mile by offering a special menu for dogs, complete with treats and non-alcoholic "pooch brews."

Dog Cafés

- Cities are increasingly opening dog cafés where you can enjoy a coffee while your dog socializes in a designated play area.

Local Delicacies

- In some cities, you can find pet bakeries offering locally-made treats that make for great souvenirs.

By incorporating these pet-friendly activities and dining options into your travel plans, you can ensure an enjoyable trip that caters to the interests of both you and your four-legged companion. Always remember to double-check specific pet policies and call ahead to confirm any details.

Safety and Health: A Comprehensive Guide to First-Aid, Handling Emergencies, and Pet Insurance

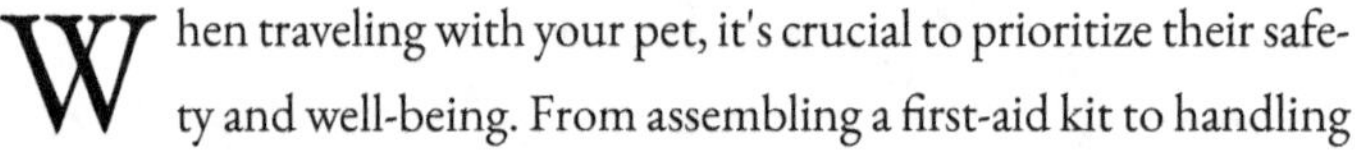

When traveling with your pet, it's crucial to prioritize their safety and well-being. From assembling a first-aid kit to handling medical emergencies and considering pet insurance, here's what you need to know to ensure a safe journey for your four-legged friend.

First-Aid Kit for Pets

Essentials

- Assemble a pet-specific first-aid kit that includes antiseptics, bandages, tweezers, and any medication your pet might need.

Pocket Guide

- Include a first-aid manual tailored for pets. Some apps also provide first-aid information and can be downloaded to your phone for quick reference.

Vet Contacts

- Keep a list of local vet services in your kit for easy access in case of emergencies.

Identification

- Update your pet's ID tag and consider including temporary tags with local contact information.

Handling Emergencies: Vet Services Abroad

Know the Nearest Vet

- Upon arrival, identify the nearest emergency veterinary service and add the contact details to your phone.

Language Barrier

- If traveling to a foreign country, learn essential veterinary terms in the local language or have them written down.

Documentation

- Always carry a copy of your pet's medical records and any important health certificates.

24-Hour Vet Services

- Find out if there is a 24-hour veterinary service in the area you're visiting. Some countries have nationwide hotlines for pet emergencies.

Pet Insurance: Do You Need It?

Coverage

- Pet insurance can cover accidents, illnesses, and even emergency vet services when you're abroad.

Pre-existing Conditions

- Check the policy details carefully. Some insurance plans don't cover pre-existing conditions.

International Coverage

- Ensure that the policy covers international travel and find out what steps you need to take to file a claim while abroad.

Cost vs. Benefits

- Weigh the cost of the insurance premium against potential out-of-pocket expenses for emergencies to determine if insurance is a worthwhile investment for your trip.

Prioritizing your pet's safety and health requires some planning and preparation but is crucial for a successful journey. With a well-stocked first-aid kit, a strategy for handling emergencies, and possibly even pet insurance, you can travel with peace of mind knowing you're prepared for almost any situation.

Parasites, Ticks, Fleas, and Climate: A Guide to Prevention, Treatment, and Comfort

♥

Travel exposes your pet to new environments and possibly to parasites like ticks and fleas, as well as varying climate conditions. It's essential to know how to prevent and treat parasitic infestations and ensure that your pet stays comfortable regardless of the weather. This guide will provide you with the necessary information to manage these aspects of your pet's health and comfort.

Parasites, Ticks, and Fleas: Prevention and Treatment

Pre-Travel Precautions

- Apply preventive flea and tick treatments before your trip. Consult your vet for recommendations based on your destination.

Regular Checks

- Perform daily checks for ticks and fleas, especially after outdoor activities.

Tools and Supplies

- Include a tick remover tool in your pet's first-aid kit. Also, pack any prescribed anti-parasite medication.

Signs of Infestation

- Know the symptoms of flea and tick-borne illnesses, such as lethargy, excessive scratching, and red or irritated skin.

Treatment

- If you find a tick, remove it carefully with the appropriate tool and consult a vet for further guidance. If a flea infestation occurs, you may need to administer medication and thoroughly clean your pet's environment.

Temperature and Climate: Keeping Your Pet Comfortable

Hot Climates

Hydration

- Always have fresh water available. Consider carrying a portable pet water bottle.

Foot Protection

- Hot pavement can burn paws. Use paw protectors or avoid walking during the hottest parts of the day.

Cooling Products

- Cooling mats, vests, and bandanas can help keep your pet

comfortable in the heat.

Cold Climates

Insulation

- Use an insulated pet bed for sleeping. Some pets may also benefit from wearing a sweater or coat.

Paw Care

- In snowy conditions, ice can build up between paw pads. Use pet-friendly ice melts and consider dog boots for extra protection.

Indoor Warmth

- Make sure your accommodation has adequate heating, and consider bringing a pet-safe space heater.

Mild Climates

- In moderate conditions, focus on providing a comfortable space for your pet with familiar blankets and bedding.

Keeping your pet free from parasites and comfortable in varying climates is integral to a successful trip. Armed with the right preventive measures, tools, and knowledge, you can ensure a healthier, happier travel experience for your furry companion.

Returning Home: Navigating Re-Entry Paperwork, Post-Travel Health, and Re-Acclimation

♥

After a journey filled with adventures and new experiences, returning home involves more than simply unpacking your bags, especially when you've traveled with a pet. The process includes navigating re-entry paperwork, making sure your pet is healthy post-travel, and helping them readjust to home life. This guide aims to provide you with a comprehensive look at what to expect and how to prepare for a smooth transition back home.

Re-Entry Paperwork and Regulations

Research in Advance

- Before you even set out on your trip, it's crucial to understand the re-entry requirements for your home country. These can vary significantly and may include quarantine periods, specific vaccinations, or even certain blood tests.

Documentation

- Always keep a well-organized file containing all relevant paperwork such as veterinary certificates, vaccination records, and any import/export permits. These documents should be easily accessible during your travel and especially upon re-entry.

Custom Declarations

- Some countries require you to declare bringing in animals at customs. Failure to comply can lead to fines or even legal trouble.

Special Requirements

- Some regions have unique regulations for specific breeds or types of animals, so make sure to comply with any additional re-entry conditions for your pet.

Digital Records

- Consider storing digital copies of all essential documents on your phone or a secure cloud service for easy access and as a backup.

Post-Travel Health Check-up

Veterinary Visit

- Schedule a post-travel check-up with your vet within a week of returning home. This visit will allow your vet to identify any potential health issues that may have arisen during the trip, such as parasites, infections, or stress-related conditions.

Monitoring

- Keep a close eye on your pet for any signs of ill-health, including lethargy, loss of appetite, or unusual behavior. Promptly consult your vet if you observe any such symptoms.

Diet Transition

- If your pet's diet changed during the trip, gradually switch them back to their regular food to avoid gastrointestinal issues.

Routine

- Resume your pet's typical exercise and feeding schedules as soon as possible. Consistency will help them readjust and alleviate any post-travel stress.

Re-Acclimating Your Pet to Home Life

The Safe Space

- Reintroduce your pet to their familiar home environment by taking them to their "safe space," whether it's a specific room, bed, or a favorite piece of furniture.

Routine Matters

- Quickly re-establish your pet's daily routine, including meals, walks, and playtime. Animals find comfort in predictability.

Social Re-Acclimation

- If you have other pets at home, reintroduce them gradually
  and under supervision to ensure there are no conflicts or
  stress.

Behavioral Changes

- Take note of any changes in your pet's behavior. Sometimes,
  pets can develop new habits or fears while traveling. If these
  changes persist, consult your vet or a pet behaviorist.

Emotional Well-being

- Spend quality time with your pet to help re-establish the
  emotional bond that might have been affected by the stresses
  of travel. A little extra attention can go a long way in helping
  your pet readjust.

Returning home with your pet involves administrative, health, and
emotional aspects that should not be overlooked. While re-entry paperwork ensures you comply with legal requirements, a post-travel
health check-up can catch any potential issues before they become
serious problems. Most importantly, helping your pet re-acclimate to
home life can go a long way in ensuring their overall well-being. All
these steps, although seemingly daunting, are integral parts of respon-

sible pet ownership and travel. With careful planning and attention to detail, you can make the transition back to everyday life as smooth as possible for both you and your pet.

Sample Packing List for Traveling with Your Pet

T raveling with your pet involves careful planning and organization, especially when it comes to packing. A comprehensive packing list can save you from last-minute stress and ensure that you have everything you need for a smooth journey. Below is a sample packing list designed to cover all the essentials and more for a hassle-free trip with your four-legged companion.

Essentials

1. **Pet Carrier** - Airline-approved if flying

2. **Leash & Collar** - Extra set is advisable

3. **Identification Tags** - Updated contact information

4. **Food & Water** - Enough for the journey plus extra

5. **Pet Bowls** - Collapsible ones save space

6. **Poop Bags or Litter Box**

7. **Basic First-Aid Kit** - Antiseptic, bandages, etc.

8. **Travel Documents** - Vaccination records, permits, etc.

9. **Prescription Medications** - If applicable

10. **Emergency Contact List** - Vets, pet care services, etc.

Comfort Items

1. **Pet Blanket or Bed** - Familiar smells can be comforting

2. **Toys** - Favorites and new ones to keep them engaged

3. **Chew Treats** - Especially useful for stressful moments

4. **Paw Wipes** - For easy cleaning on-the-go

5. **Grooming Supplies** - Brush, pet-safe shampoo, etc.

Food & Hydration

1. **Sealable Food Containers** - Keeps food fresh

2. **Travel Water Bottle** - With a built-in bowl

3. **Snacks** - Treats and chewable to keep them busy

4. **Can Opener** - If you're packing canned food

Health & Safety

1. **Tick/Flea Preventatives**

2. **Sunscreen** - Pet-safe formula

3. **Cooling Mat** - For hot climates

4. **Paw Protectors** - For extreme temperatures or rough terrain

5. **Reflective Gear** - Leash/collar for visibility

Extras

1. **Camera** - For capturing memories

2. **GPS Tracker** - For added safety

3. **Calming Aids** - Sprays, wraps, or diffusers for anxious pets

4. **Pet Stroller or Wagon** - For when they get tired

5. **Portable Pen or Play Area** - Useful for outdoor settings

Before you start packing, consider your destination, the length of your stay, and your planned activities. This will help you tailor this packing list to your specific needs. Remember, the key to a successful trip is preparation, so start packing well in advance and double-check your list before you head out the door. Safe travels!

Useful Websites and Apps for Traveling with Your Pet

♥

Planning a trip with your pet can be a challenging task, but luckily, there are various online resources and apps designed to make the process easier. Here's a list of useful websites and mobile applications to help you plan a seamless journey with your furry companion.

Websites

Pet Travel Services

1. **PetTravel.com** - Comprehensive information on airline

policies, pet-friendly hotels, and other services.

2. **BringFido.com** - Allows you to search for dog-friendly activities, eateries, and accommodations around the world.

Health and Safety

1. **AVMA.org (American Veterinary Medical Association)** - Reliable advice on travel safety and health tips.

2. **CDC.gov** - The Centers for Disease Control and Prevention offer guidelines on traveling with pets internationally.

Booking Platforms

1. **Booking.com (Pet-friendly filter)** - Accommodation search with an option to filter pet-friendly stays.

2. **Airbnb (Pets Allowed filter)** - Many listings indicate whether pets are allowed.

Forums and Blogs

1. **Reddit's r/pets** - A place to ask for travel advice specific to your pet's needs.

2. **The Dogington Post** - Offers dog-specific travel tips and product reviews.

Apps

Trip Planning

1. **BringFido** (iOS/Android) - Find pet-friendly locations and services on the go.

2. **Pawtrack** (iOS/Android) - Collar with a GPS that lets you monitor your cat's whereabouts.

Health and Safety

1. **Pet First Aid** (iOS/Android) - Developed by the American Red Cross, it provides veterinary advice for everyday emergencies.

2. **VitusVet** (iOS/Android) - Keep your pet's medical records in one place, making it easier during vet visits, especially on the road.

Activity Trackers

1. **Whistle** (iOS/Android) - GPS and activity monitor to keep track of your pet's location and exercise levels.

2. **FitBark** (iOS/Android) - An activity tracker that monitors your pet's movements and provides insights into their behavior and health.

Misc

1. **Pet Care Services** (iOS/Android) - Find nearby pet care services like dog walkers, pet sitters, and more.

2. **iKibble** (iOS/Android) - Quick reference guide for what foods are safe for dogs to eat.

Before relying heavily on any website or app, remember to check reviews or recommendations for reliability. Always consult professionals for medical or legal advice. These tools are meant to supplement your own research and preparation for a well-planned and safe journey with your pet.

Resources for Further Reading: Expanding Your Knowledge on Traveling with Pets

♥

If you're looking to dive deeper into the world of pet travel, numerous resources can offer you more detailed information, tips, and insights. Below is a list of various types of resources that are worth exploring for anyone interested in becoming an expert on traveling with pets.

**Books

1. **"The Dog Lover's Guide to Travel" by Kelly E. Carter** - Offers tips on pet-friendly hotels, restaurants, and attractions across North America.

2. **"On the Road with Your Pet" by Dawn and Robert Habgood** - A comprehensive guide to car travel with your pet, covering everything from safety to comfort.

3. **"Pet Travel: A Guide to the Journey" by Sandra Hanks** - An all-encompassing manual on how to travel safely and happily with your pet, both domestically and internationally.

Academic Journals and Papers

1. **"Travel-induced stress in dogs: behavior and physiological effects"** - A research paper that delves into the science behind travel-related stress in dogs.

2. **"The Importance of Pet Travel Safety"** - A scholarly article focusing on the legal and ethical responsibilities of traveling with pets.

Online Blogs and Articles

1. **The Points Paws** - A sub-section of the popular blog The Points Guy, focusing on pet travel tips and hacks.

2. **GoPetFriendly Blog** - Provides a wealth of articles covering everything from packing lists to destination guides for pet

owners.

3. **PetTravelTales.com** - Personal experiences and advice from seasoned pet travelers.

Podcasts

1. **"Pet Life Radio — Take Meow-t to the Ball Game"** - Offers episodes on traveling with pets, including interviews with veterinarians and travel experts.

2. **"The Woof Life Show"** - Focuses on various pet topics, including episodes about pet travel.

Webinars and Online Courses

1. **"Preparing Your Pet for Travel"** - A webinar offered by various pet travel agencies that guide you through the preparations needed for safe pet travel.

2. **"Pet First Aid & CPR"** - Online courses to equip you with the skills needed to handle emergencies while traveling with your pet.

Social Media Groups

1. **Facebook Groups like "Traveling with Dogs" or "Cat Explorers"** - Community advice and real-world experiences from other pet owners who travel.

2. **Instagram Hashtags like #PetTravel or #Travel-ingWithPets** - Offers visual ideas and inspiration for pet-friendly destinations and activities.

By exploring these resources, you can broaden your understanding of what it means to travel with a pet, ensuring that both you and your four-legged companion have the best experience possible.

www.ingramcontent.com/pod-product-compliance
Lightning Source LLC
Chambersburg PA
CBHW070904260726

48661CB00004B/1596